Introducing ... YOUR AMYGDALA

Oh my gosh you're here! I'm your amygdala, and I'm so excited to meet you. I've actually known you since you were born (kid, you were adorable - still are), but now you can get to know me properly. Let me introduce myself.

I'm kind of fabulous. My job is to protect you, and I'm brilliant at it. Sometimes a little too brilliant. I just want to keep you safe, so sometimes I can be a little overprotective - I might worry you're in danger when actually it's just you, being epic, doing something brave. You see, I can't always tell the difference between two very different kinds of 'scary':

SCARY-SAFE (brave, challenging, or new things)

SCARY-DANGEROUS (things that could actually hurt you)

I need your help to tell the difference.

You and me - we're the dream team, kid. My job is to do the worrying for us. Yours is to do the calming. This book will show you how. All complicated, beautiful things make sense when there are a few good instructions, and I'm no different. Ready kid? Let's get to know me.

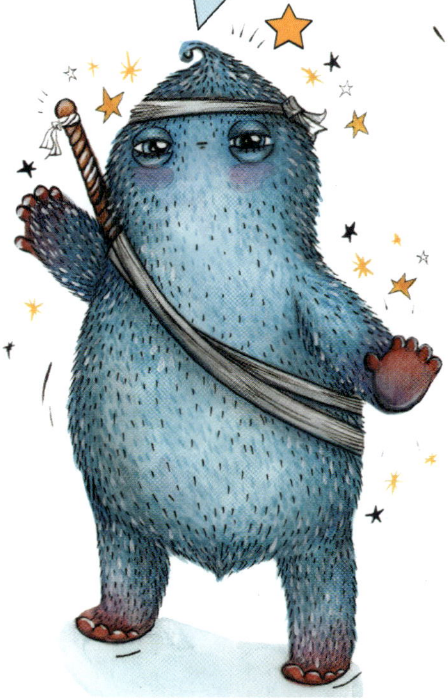

My amygdala ROCKS

Here's a very lovely and sometimes annoying truth: **brave things ALWAYS come with anxiety.** It's the anxiety that makes them brave. Want some proof? Let's break it down.

What's something you've done that was brave?

How did you feel just before it?

How did you feel just after?

Have you heard of the BRAVE SPACE?

The space between 'BEFORE BRAVE' and 'I DID IT!' is the 'BRAVE SPACE'. Brave rarely feels like 'brave'. It might actually feel more like ...

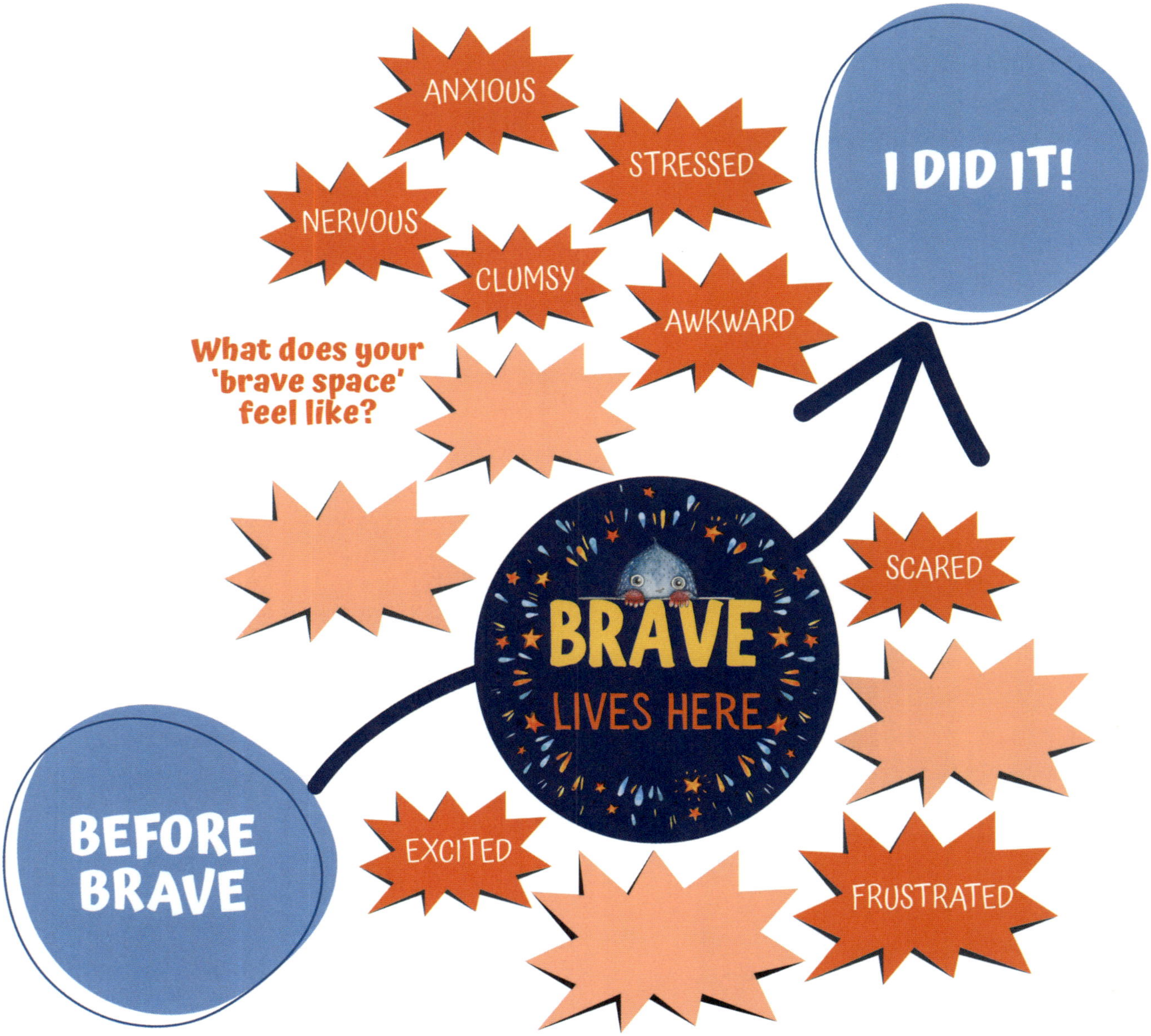

'Brave' happens in the brave space.
It's about DOING brave, even when you don't FEEL brave.

Two ways to move through the BRAVE SPACE

1. Two Questions.

Just because something feels scary, doesn't mean it's dangerous or bad for you. Mostly, it means you're about to do something brave or something that matters.

When something feels scary or hard, ask yourself:

Do I feel like this because I'm in danger,
or because there's something brave, hard, new, or important I need to do?

then,

Is this a time for me to be safe, or is this a time for me to be brave?

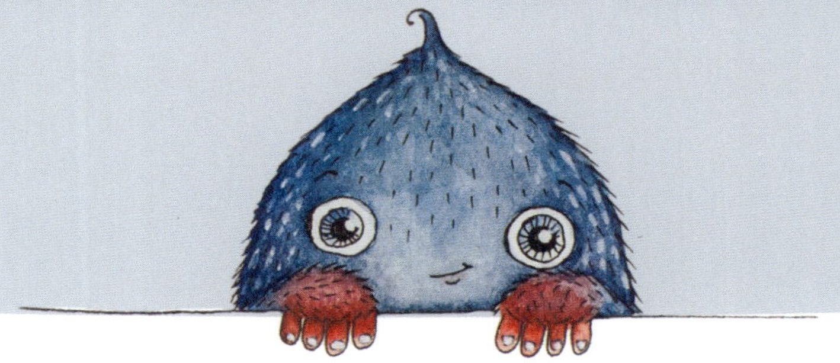

2. How to turn anxiety into excitement ... 'ANXCITEMENT'

Anxcited. Yep. It's a thing - a mix of '**I'm anxious**' and '**This could be amazing!**' Here's a zingy little brain gem for you: Anxiety and excitement are the same in your body (racey heart, fluttery tummy - you know how it goes), but they feel different because of what you focus on. It's all about where you point the spotlight.

When you focus on what could go wrong, you'll feel anxious.
When you focus on what could go right, you'll feel excited.

Next time your amygdala gets anxious because it's spotlighting all the risks, help it shift into *anxcited* (maybe even excited - all excitement, no anxiety!) by asking yourself:

What if this actually turns out better than I imagined?
How would I feel? What good things might happen?

Write your answer, and keep it close. Focus on it when you're in the brave space.

Anxiety is just excitement that forgot how fabulous you are. Time to remind it.
You've got this, legend.

Let's get to know me!

Like all fabulous important things (you're one of them, kid), I need a name. I mean, 'Amygdala' is nice, it's classic, but a bit, you know, common. So go for it.
What are we going to call me?

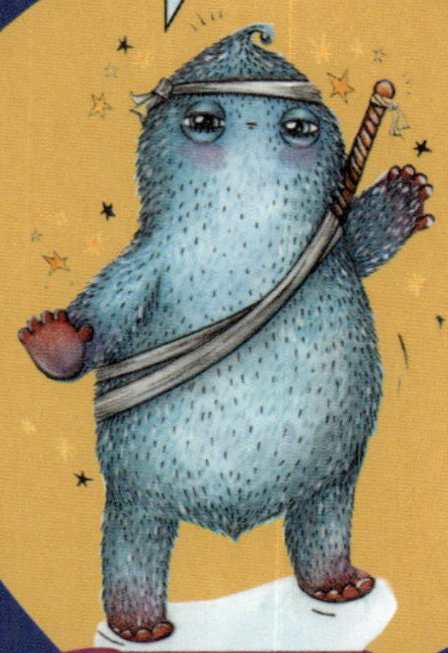

SOMETHING TO TRY:
The yeps and the nopes.

Inside the amygdala shape, write or draw the things that upset your amygdala. What makes it anxious, sad, or angry? Which are **scary-safe**? Which are **scary-dangerous**? **Outside** the shape, write or draw the things that help your amygdala feel calm, safe, and happy.

SOMETHING ELSE:
A cut-out.

Use the template to cut an amygdala shape from felt or cardboard. Now zhuzh it up with anything you like - paint, sequins, a smidge of bubble wrap, a handy pocket for emergency snacks or sunshine. Anything.

ANOTHER OPTION: A plushie.
(Awww cute ...a 'me' you can hug!)

Use the template to cut the amygdala shape from fabric. Next, flip that fabric over like a pancake (but don't eat it!) and cut another amygdala shape. Now you have the front and back of your amygdala. Time to stitch things up! Sew the pieces together, but before you seal the deal with your final stitch, stuff your amygdala bud with cushion stuffing.

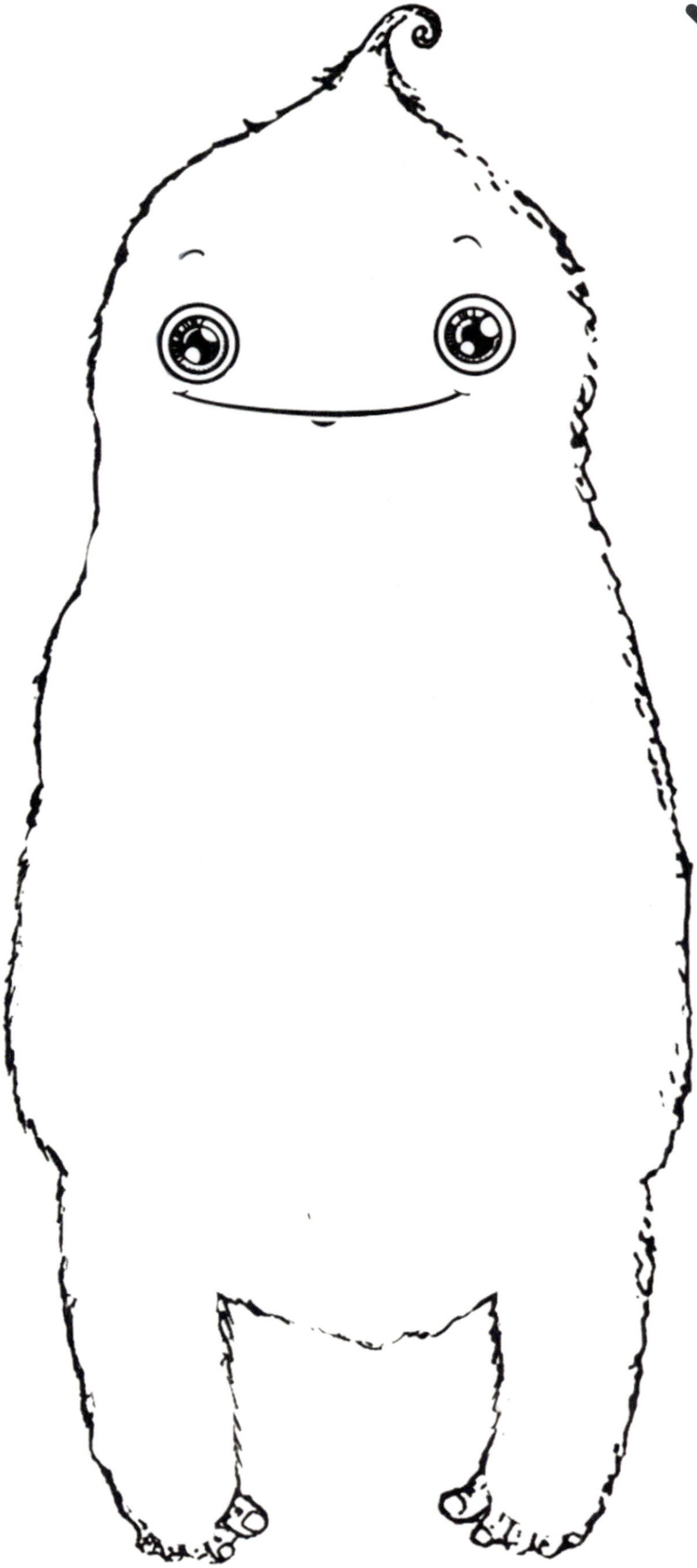

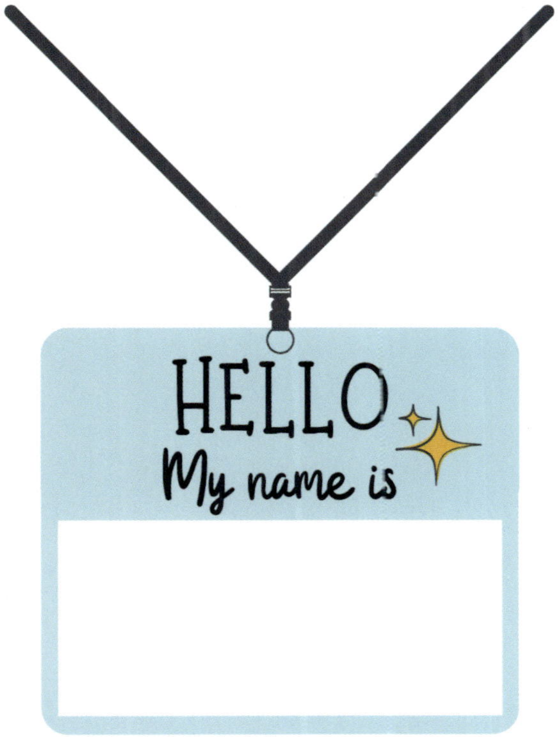
HELLO
My name is

During anxiety, ALL bodies can get ...

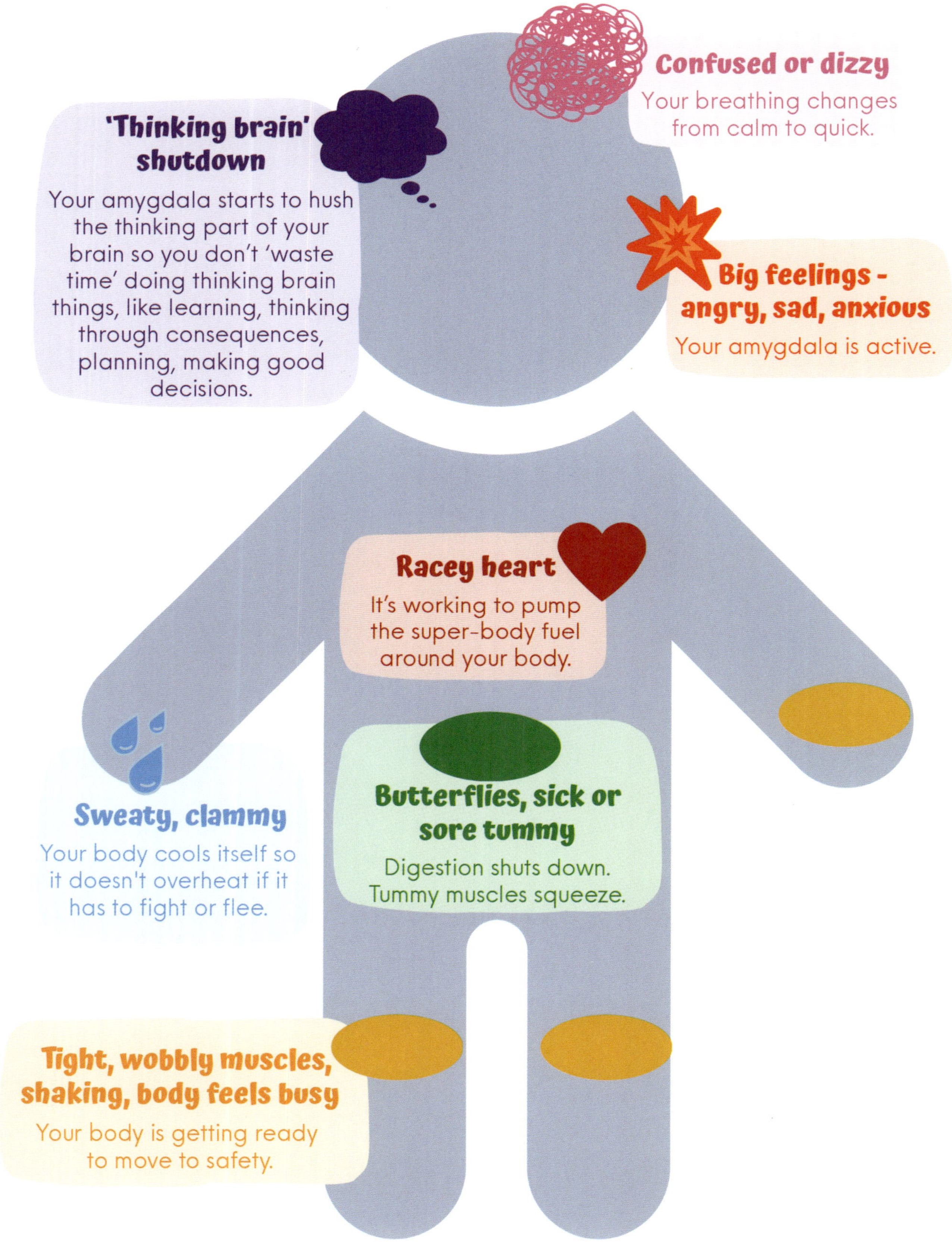

What happens in YOUR body?

The House Model

There are three ways your brain and body work to protect you. Think of this like a three-level house.

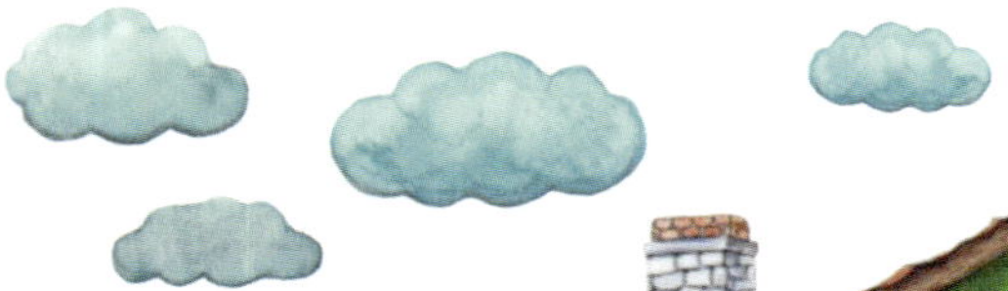

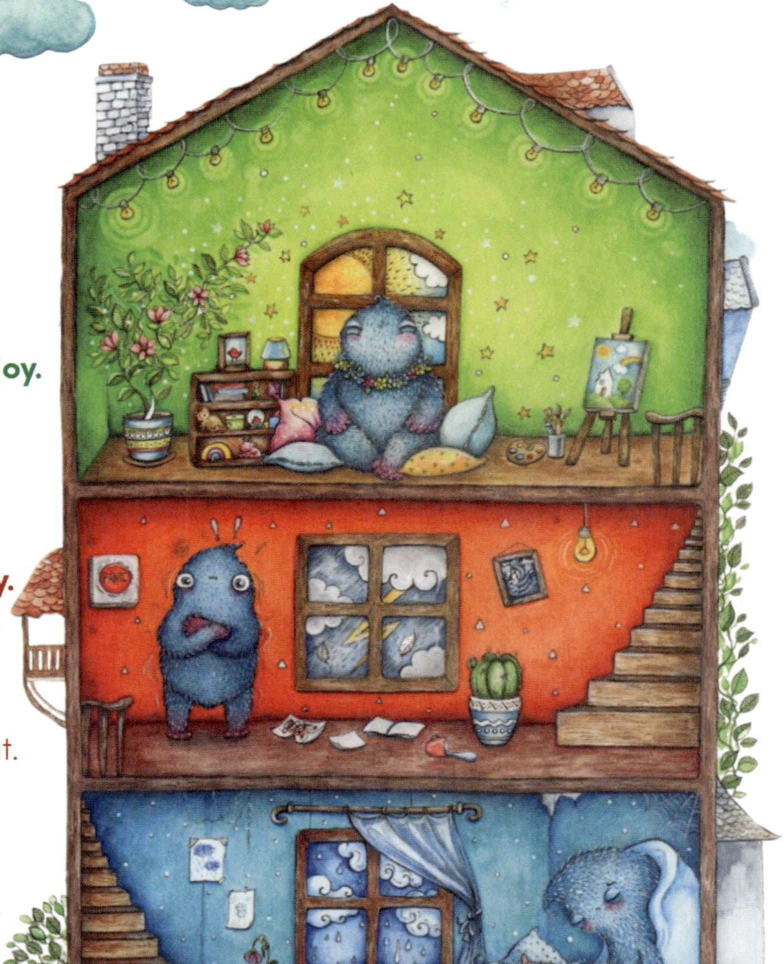

On the top floor

My body feels calm.
I feel happy, relaxed.
I can learn, play, connect, feel joy.

My amygdala feels safe.

On the middle floor

My body feels busy, active, fizzy.
I feel anxious, irritated, angry, agitated, frustrated.

My brain and body are working to get me safe through movement.

On the bottom floor

My body feels still, tired, heavy.
I feel helpless, hopeless, sad, withdrawn.

My brain and body are working to keep me safe by hiding or being small and still.

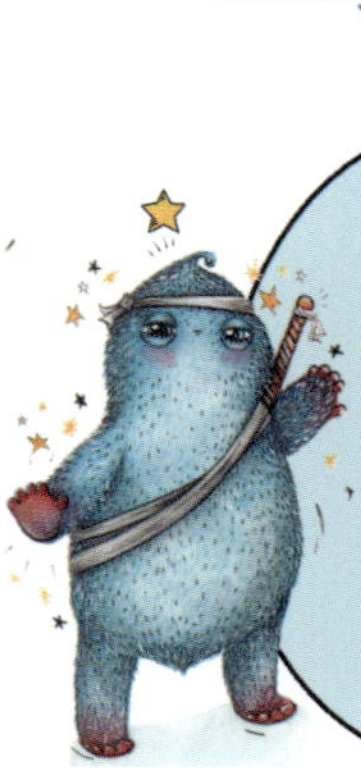

Ok, kid – we need to talk about calm breathing ... It's one of the most powerful ways to get to 'top-level calm' – **but it takes practice**. If you've tried it when you're upset and it doesn't work, it's because you haven't done it enough when you're calm. Even though you've been breathing your whole life (love that about you), breathing is usually automatic. Your brain takes care of it while you're busy being fabulous. To calm me down, you need to 'breathe on purpose': slow, steady, and in charge.

On the TOP FLOOR ...

I feel happy and safe.

My amygdala is calm. My body feels relaxed. I might feel like playing or hanging out with myself or people who feel good to be around.

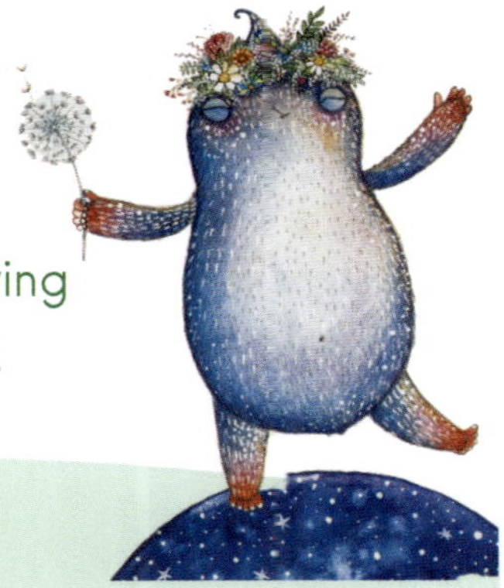

When do you feel like this?

What do you feel in your body? What thoughts are you aware of?

What helps you stay here? What do you enjoy doing? Who are the people who feel good to be around, or the places that feel good to be?

What do adults do (or what would you like them to do) to help you feel cared for?

On the MIDDLE FLOOR...

I feel anxious, angry, irritated, frustrated.
My amygdala is panicked. My body feels too busy. It might feel like it needs to move fast, run, pace, or wriggle, or as though it has hits, kicks, or spicy words in it that want to come out.

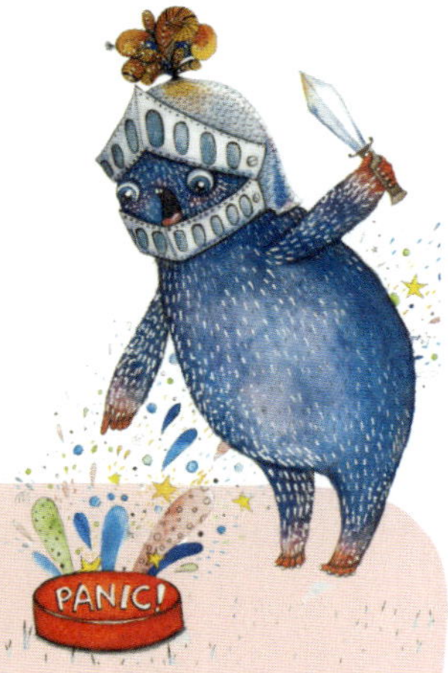

When have you felt like this? What takes you here?

What do you feel in your body? What thoughts are you aware of?

What can help you get back to the top floor? What's helped in the past?

What makes it hard to get back to top-level calm sometimes?

What can the adults around you do that would help, or not make it worse?

On the BOTTOM FLOOR ...

I feel sad, hopeless, helpless, still, numb.
My body feels heavy, tired, slumped. Sometimes I feel as though I want to hide or be away from everyone and everything.

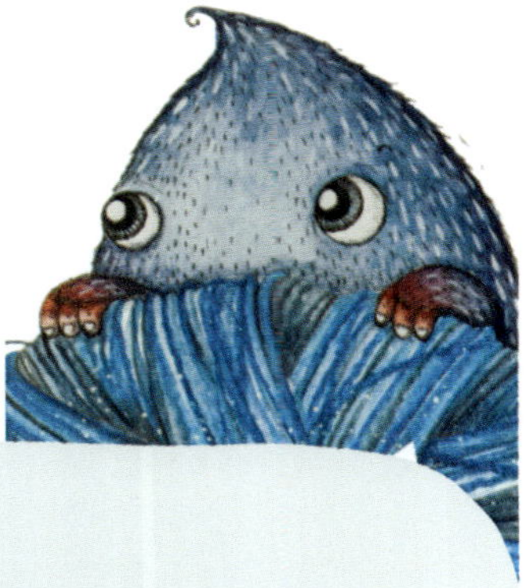

When have you felt like this? What takes you here?

What do you feel in your body? What thoughts are you aware of?

What can help you get back to the top floor? What's helped in the past?

What makes it hard to get back to top-level calm sometimes?

What can the adults around you do that would help, or not make it worse?

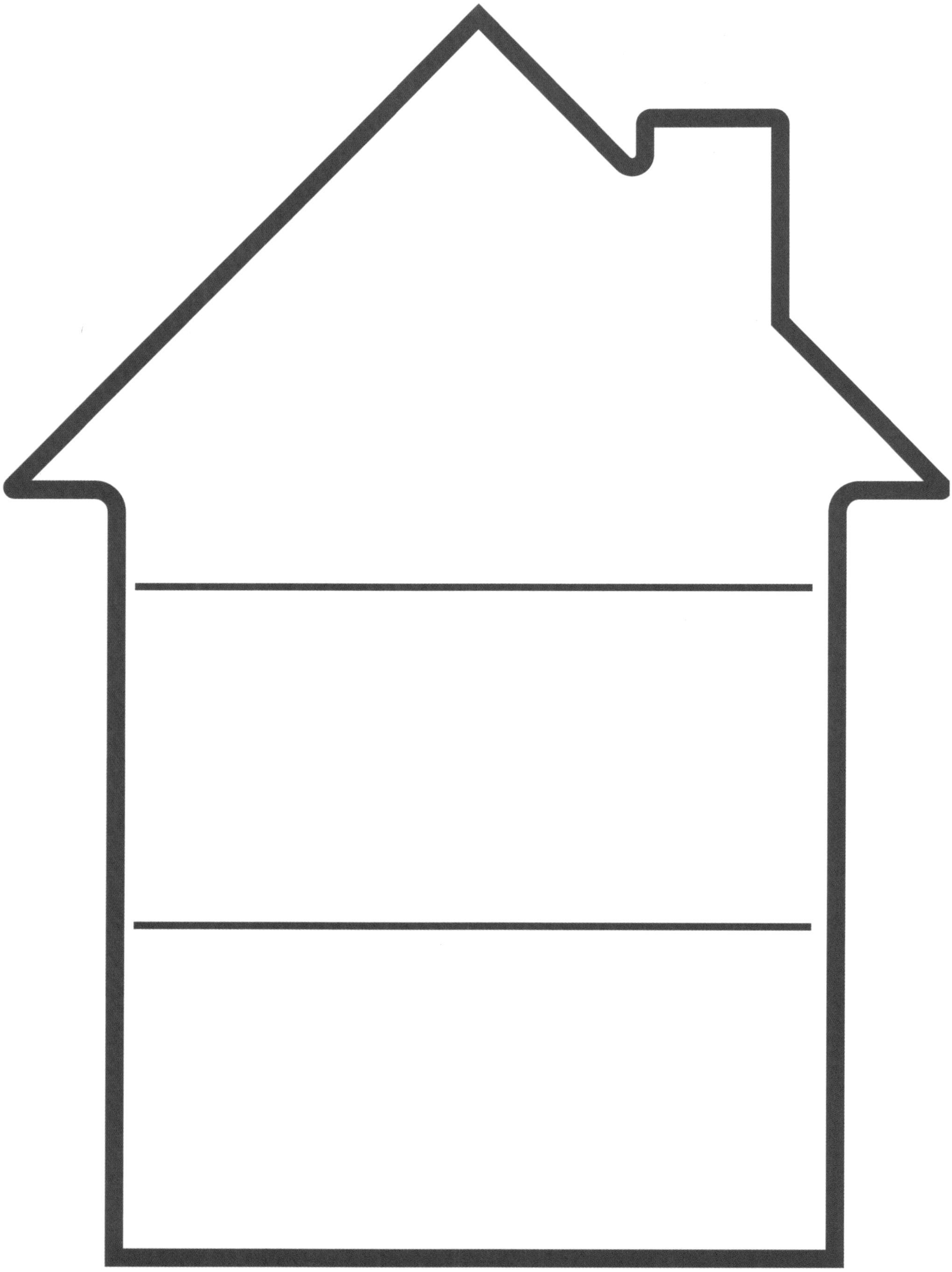

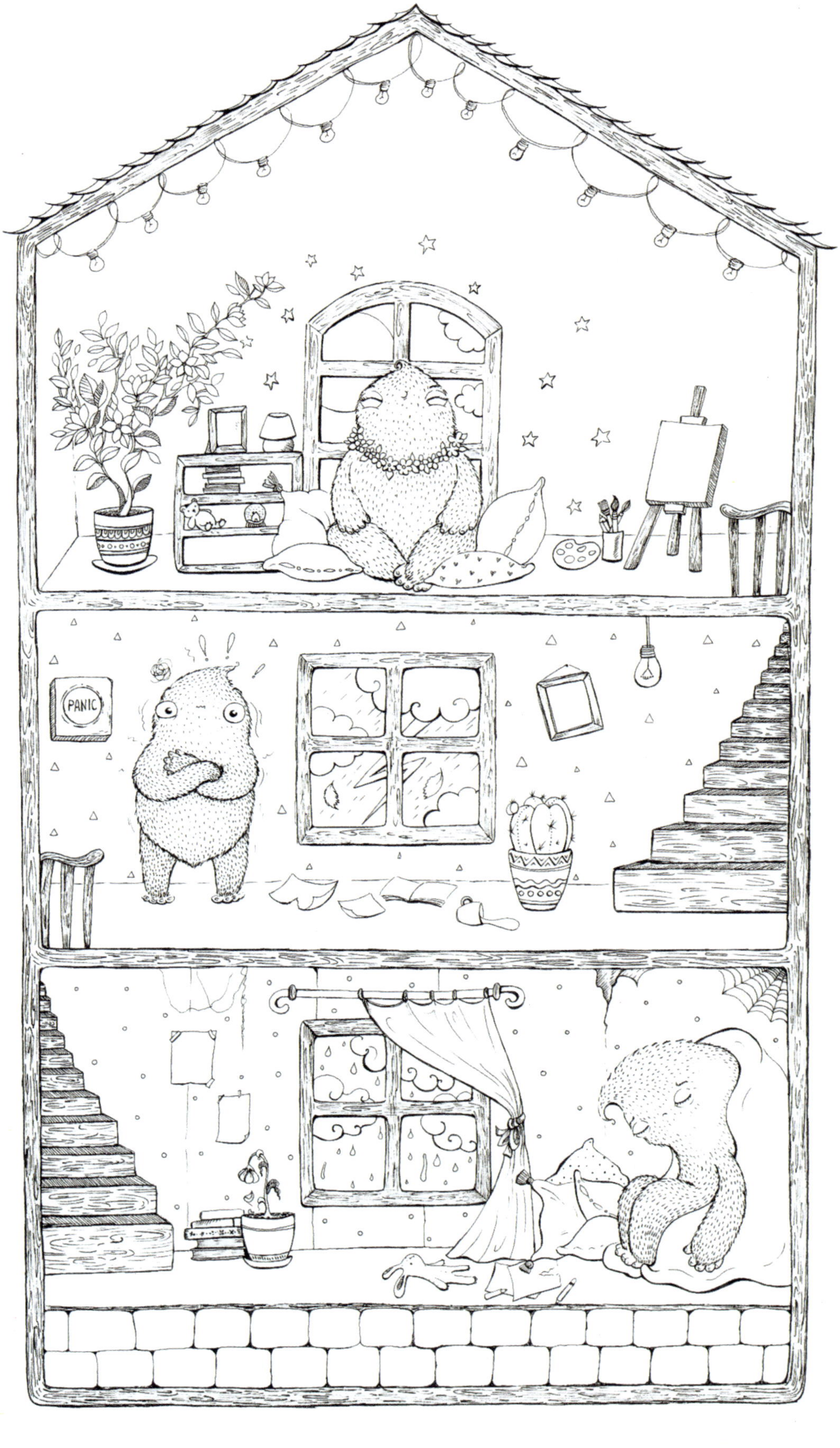

Here's a photo of me. I love this photo. The photographer had snacks. Cut out the photo and pop some velcro or blu-tack on the back, then take me up and down the levels to show how you're feeling.

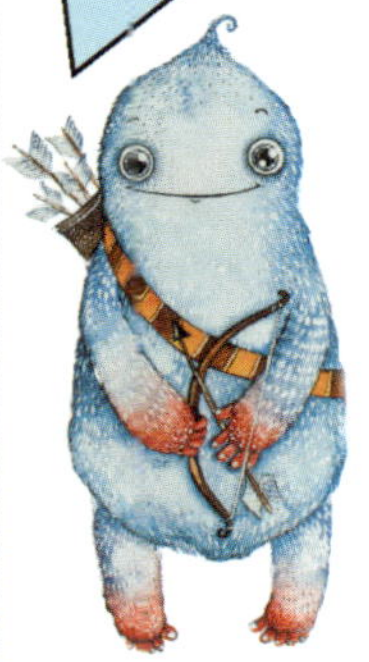

Okay, legend: Some brain science for you.

Your brain has two main parts. In the back is your **'feeling brain'**. This is where your amygdala lives. Up front is the **'thinking brain'**. They need to work together, like co-pilots, so you can feel your feelings **and** make good decisions. But when your amygdala gets upset, your **feeling brain** takes over and your **thinking brain** ducks out for a nap: 'Dude, I'm out. Call me when things calm down.' (It doesn't actually say this though, because brains can't talk - no lips.)

Without your thinking brain as co-pilot, things can get messy. Fast. (We've all been there!) The more upset your amygdala is (the bigger your feelings), the harder it is to think clearly. There are no wrong feelings, but you need to be the boss of your amygdala. Feel your feelings (go ahead - have a moment!), but make sure your thinking brain is on board.

A PAPER MACHE BRAIN MODEL (Or a hat. That's right. A hat. For your brain.)

What you need:

- a balloon, blown up to about the size of your fabulous head
- plain paper
- a paintbrush
- glue (Or make your own: Mix equal parts flour and water. Stir until there are no lumps. Add a few spoons of salt to stop it going gross.)

What to do:

- Tear the paper into wild little strips and soak them in the glue.
- Cover the balloon with 2-3 layers of paper. Let it dry completely, then go again with 2-3 more layers.
- When it's dry, pop the balloon with a needle and cut the paper mache ball in half.
- Decorate the back half as your feeling brain and the front half as your thinking brain.

To turn it into a brain hat:

- Poke a little hole on either side and thread some elastic through so it won't fly off mid-cartwheel.
- Ok - this is your moment. Stand in front of a mirror. Put it on - same place crowns go. Hello there fancy head!

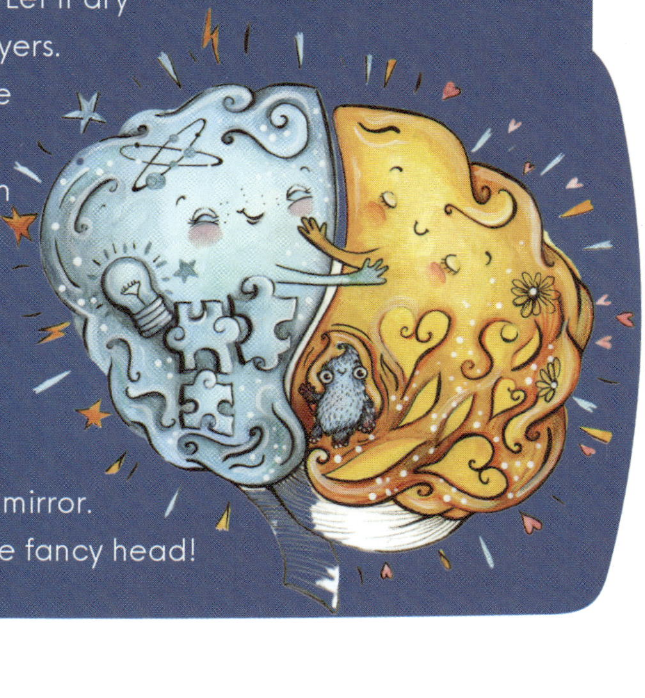

It's hard to think clearly sometimes!

Understanding the relationship between your feeling brain and thinking brain.

A GLITTER JAR

What you'll need:

- glitter glue
- a clear glass jar or plastic bottle with a lid
- warm water

What to do:

- Fill the jar or bottle with warm water.
- Add a few big drops of glitter glue.
- Replace the lid and shake.
- Imagine the glitter is your thoughts. Now shake the jar. See the stormy chaos? This is what happens when your feelings get big. Can you see clearly? Nope. Can you think straight? Nuh-uh. Now, watch what happens when you're still for a few moments. Just watch and breathe. See how the glitter storm (feelings storm) starts to settle? Now you're back in business: thinking straight, seeing straight, straight-up legend.

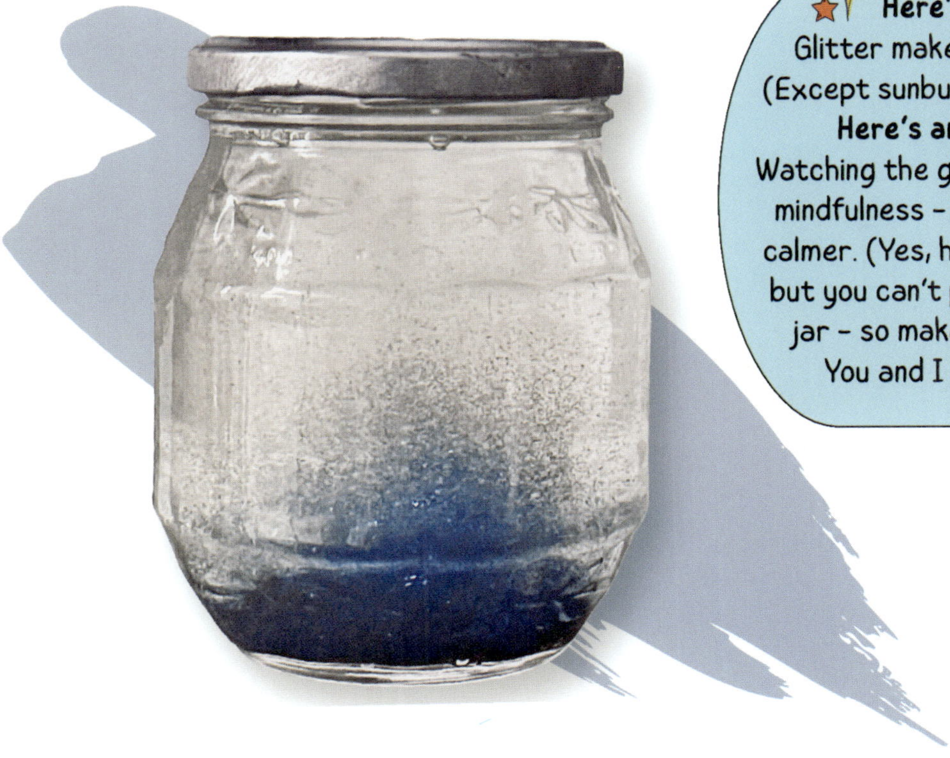

Here's a handy tip:
Glitter makes everything lovelier.
(Except sunburn, but you knew that.)
Here's another handy tip:
Watching the glitter settle is an act of mindfulness – it will help us both feel calmer. (Yes, holidays will do that too, but you can't put a holiday in a handy jar – so make us a glitter jar, kid. You and I will love you for it.)

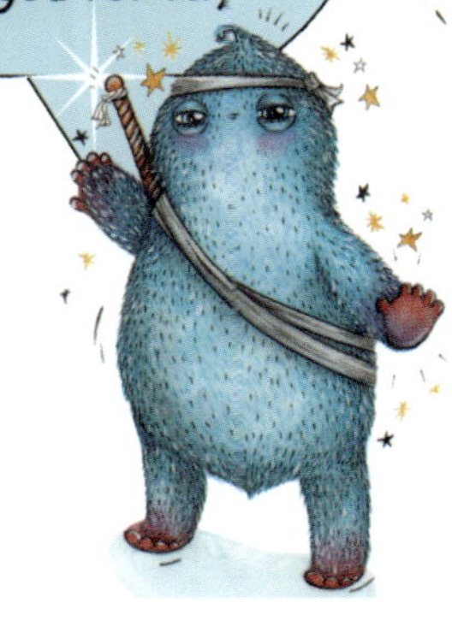

Create your CALM SPACE.

Why it works:

Thoughts are hefty little powerhouses. They can change how you feel and what you do. A clever way to use this brainpower to feel calmer is by creating your very own 'perfect-for-you' space to go to in your imagination when you feel anxious. When you imagine feeling safe and calm, your brain and body will follow. (Brains and bodies are so clever like that.)

What to do:

- Imagine a place where you feel safe, happy, and calm. Draw it, paint it, write about it, or hold it in your imagination. It might be somewhere you've been, somewhere you've seen, or somewhere you create. It can be anything you like - a treehouse, a magic carpet, a swing on a faraway star, a sun-kissed beach, a cloud hammock in the sky, a giant bubble that floats you wherever you want to go. Now explore your special place, especially through your senses.

  - **Where is your special place?**
  - **What do you see, smell, hear, feel when you are there?**
  - **What's the weather like? Is it warm and inviting? Cool and refreshing?**
  - **How does your body feel when you are there?**
  - **What or who is there with you? Pets? People? Magical creatures? Favourite things? Just you?**

- Think about how you get to your special place.

  - **Do you close your eyes and imagine yourself there? Are there words or actions that help with this? What do you feel in your body as you do this?**
  - **Do you fly there? With wings? In a hot air balloon? A helicopter? On a friendly dragon called Sheldon? What do you hear? See? Feel?**
  - **Do you ride there? On a bike? Glide there on the back of a whale? How do these look, sound, feel?**
  - **Do you walk, run, swim, swing, skate there? Climb there on a moonlit staircase?**

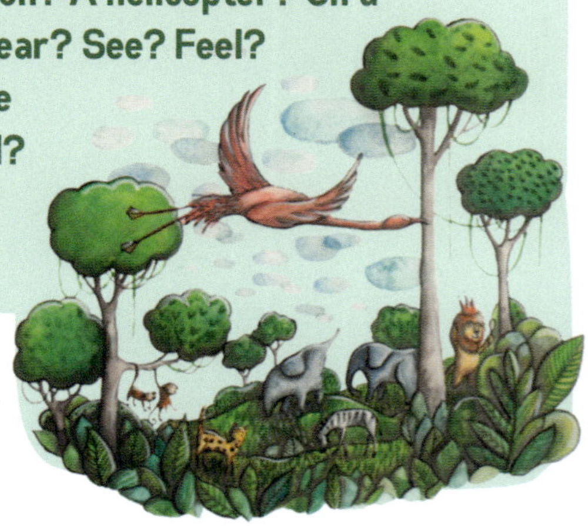

- Each day, spend a few minutes imagining yourself in your special place so it's easier to take yourself there when you want to.

MY SPECIAL PLACE

**Write about, paint, or draw your special place.
Remember, this is *your* place to go to when you want some calm, some happy, or a little bit of magic. It can be anything you want it to be.**

The POWER TOOLS

Powerful ways to calm your amygdala and switch on your thinking brain..

GROUNDING

Why it works:

Anxiety is all about 'what if'. Grounding brings your brain back to 'what is'. Brains feel safest in the present because right now, right here, they are safe. Sometimes they just need to be shown the way. Grounding lets you do this.

What to do:

As you breathe, notice:

- 5 things you can see
- 4 things you can feel outside your body
- 3 things you can hear
- 2 things you can smell
- 1 thing you can taste

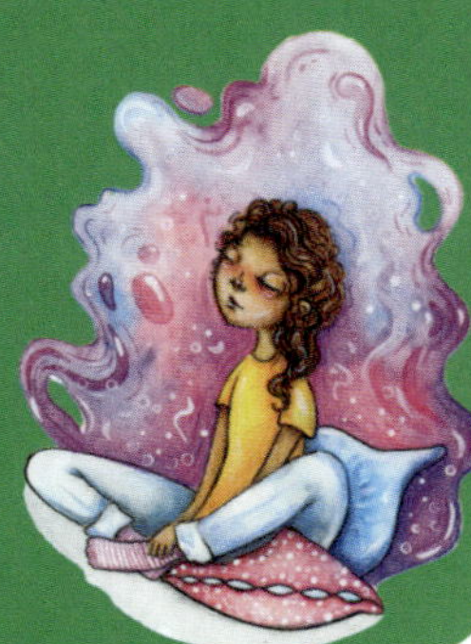

COLD WATER SPLASH

Why it works:

In your body is a very powerful, very long pair of nerves called the vagus nerve. They're like brakes for your big feelings. Cold water turns on the brakes to calm your amygdala (and your big feels).

What to do:

Splash cold water onto your face, or hold an icepack against your face or the back of your neck.

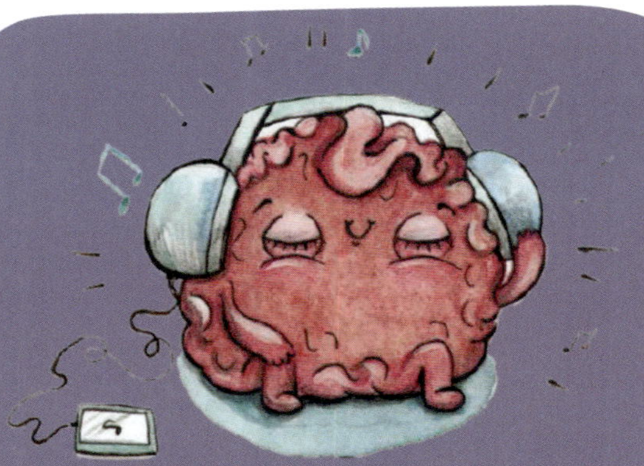

HUMMING

Why it works:

Brains feel safe when you're humming, because we can't hum unless we feel safe. (When was the last time you hummed while you were running from a bear? Not a teddy bear - a grizzly one that threw chips at you.) It's a quick trick to remind your brain that you're okay.

What to do:

Hum - there's no wrong way to do it!

MOVEMENT

Why it works:

When there's no danger and no need to move, there's nothing to burn the super-body fuel surging through you. This is completely safe, but it can feel awful. Movement will help burn this fuel and calm your body.

What to do:

Walk, run, kick a ball, dance, do wall push-ups, shake, skip, swing your arms from side to side or front to back.

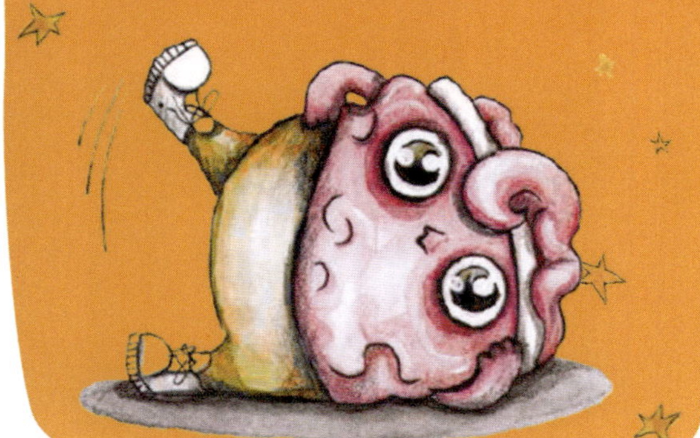

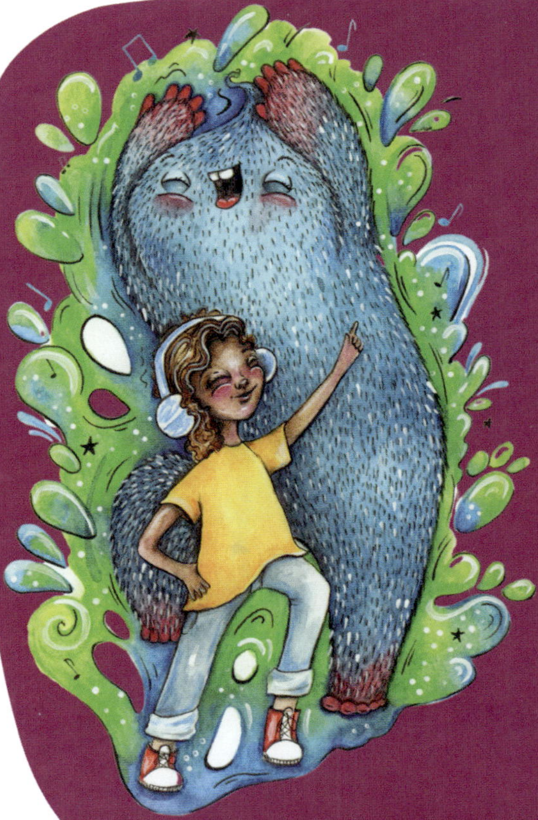

RHYTHM

Why it works:

Rhythm helps brains feel safe and calm. Whether it's the steady beat of a drum or the gentle sway of a lullaby, brains adore rhythm.

What to do:

Body Drumming - Drum a rhythm against your body in time to music. Use your hands against your thighs, arms, knees, chest, or clap them together. Search 'body percussion' online to find lots of routines, or make up your own!

Other ways to use rhythm to feel calm:

- Listen/drum/tap/stomp to music.
- Sway, swing, dance.
- Sit in a rocking chair.
- Create a playlist with a rhythm that you can walk fast or run to.

SPAGHETTI BODIES

This is how relaxed feels!

Why it works:

When anxiety hangs around for a while, your body can forget what 'relaxed' feels like. This can make you feel tense without even noticing. Here's the kicker: when your body is tense, your brain will be too. Your brain follows your body - **but** (and here's the good bit) it also works the other way. Relax your body, and your brain will follow, calm and cruisy. Bit tricky? Totally. Bit genius? Also totally.

What to do:

Imagine you are a hard strand of uncooked spaghetti. Make your body super tense and stiff. Hold this for a few seconds, then go super floppy, like wobbly cooked spaghetti. Shake and wobble for a few seconds. Now, tense your body again like raw spaghetti. Hold, then loosen again. Repeat this 4 or 5 times.

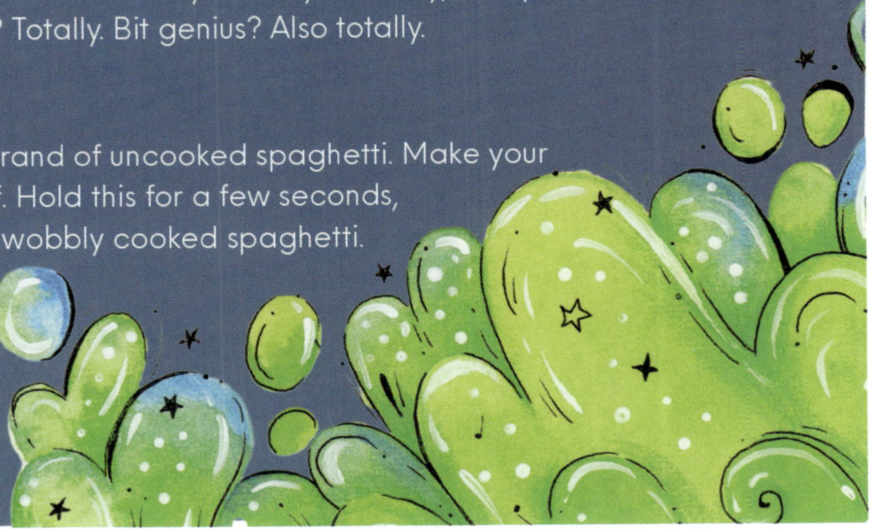

SHAKE IT OUT

Why it works:

With each wiggle, jiggle, and shake, you'll gently release any stress and anxiety that might be held in your body. Your amygdala will love you for it.

What to do:

Version 1: Shake and Halve

- Shake your right hand 16 times while counting quickly to 16. Repeat with your left hand (16 shakes), right hand (16 shakes), left leg (16 shakes), right leg (16 shakes), and hips (16 side to side).
- Now say, 'Halve it!' and repeat the sequence, but shake 8 times - arms, legs, hips.
- Then say 'Halve it!' and repeat the sequence with 4 shakes, then 2 shakes, then 1.

Version 2: Shake and Sound

- Shake your left arm 10 times. Repeat with your right arm, left leg, right leg.
- Now shake your whole body, as gently or as fast as you like. As you do this, let out any noises inside you. This might even sound like a roar!

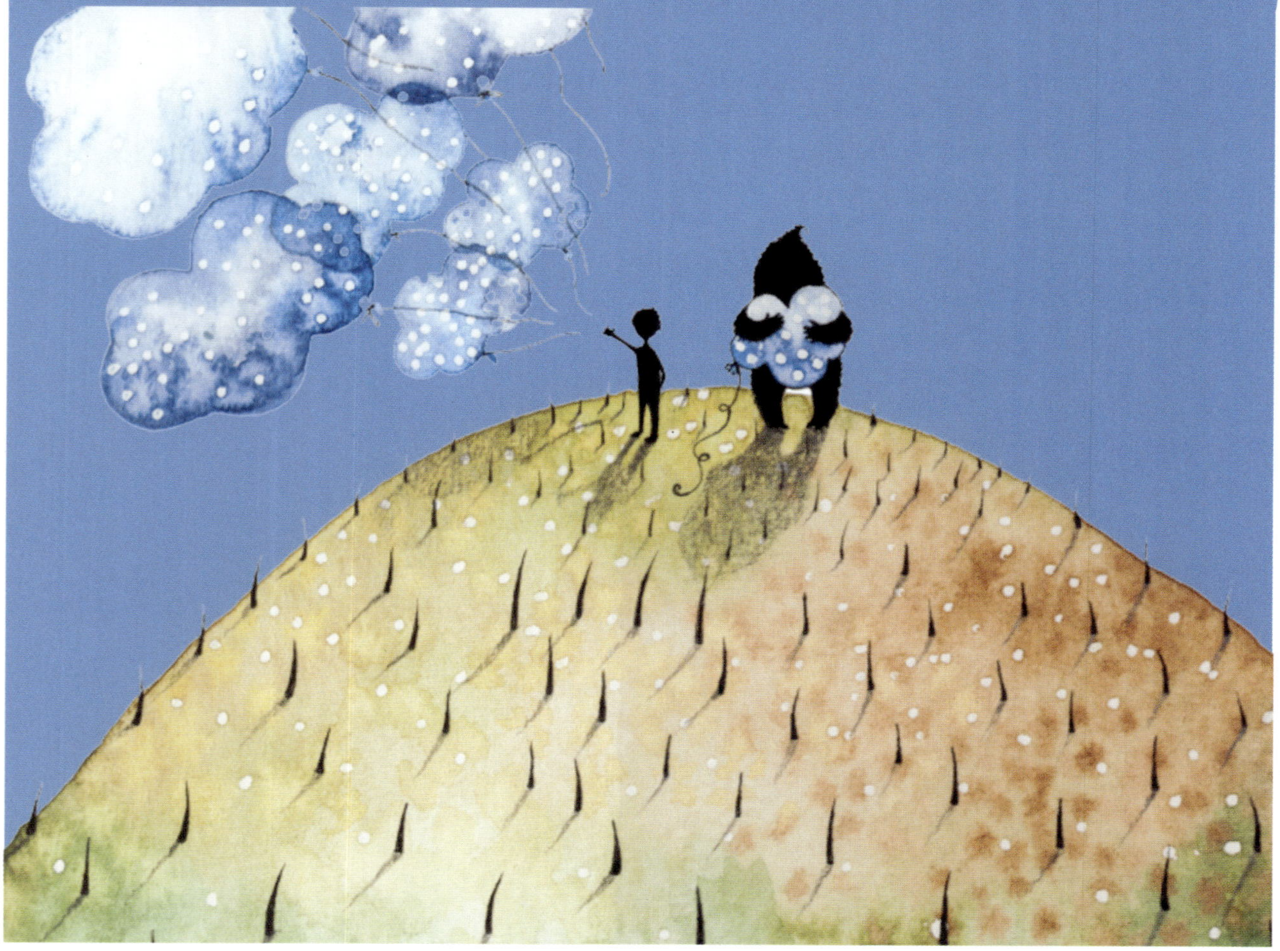

WHERE DOES YOUR 'BRAVE' LIVE?

Why it works:

We all have a brave part that lives inside us. Let's find that part in you.

What to do:

Get comfy and take three strong, deep belly breaths. Let your breath fill your belly like a balloon. (If you're not a fan of deep breathing, slow and steady works brilliantly too.) If you want to, close your eyes for an extra calming touch. On your next breath, imagine where inside you your 'brave' lives. It might be in your head, your chest, your heart, your belly, or your little toe. There are no wrong answers. If you aren't sure where it lives, can you guess? Now, put your hand over it. As you breathe, imagine that brave part of you getting bigger and bigger, and moving closer and closer to your hand with every breath. After a few slow breaths, imagine that your 'brave' is so big and so close now you can almost touch it. That brave part of you has something to say. Let's hear it.

- What would it say if it could talk?
- Draw the picture or write the words that came from that brave part of you.

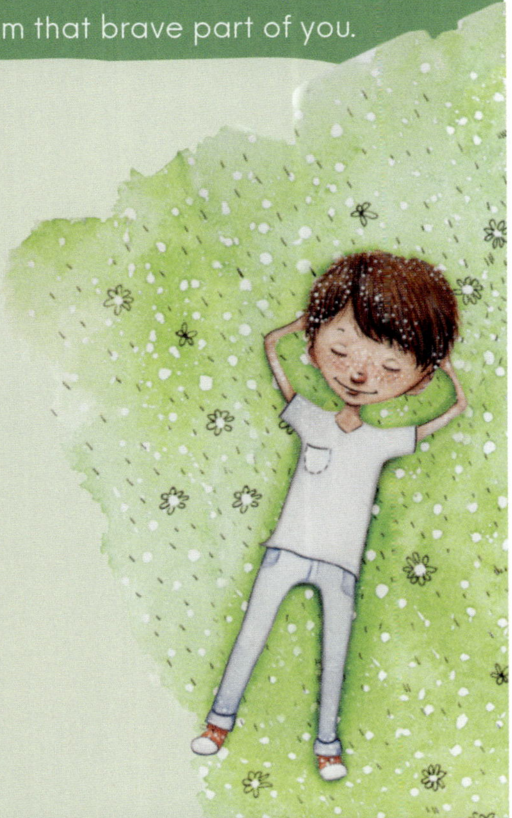

You might want to ...

Use these words as a mantra (something you say over and over to yourself) when you are doing your calm breathing, or use the words or picture as a 'bravery power-up' when you need to feel stronger, braver and more powerful.

CALM BREATHING

The MOST POWERFUL way to be the boss of your amygdala.

Why it works:

Calm, slow breathing is like a sweet, sweet lullaby for an amygdala. But when your brain is swirling with big feelings, it gets too busy to remember new moves like 'breathing on purpose'. That's why it's important to practice when you're calm. Here are some breathing exercises to try. Pick the ones you like most and practice for a few minutes a day.

STOP and feel your breathing.

Think of your breath like an anchor. You can use it any time to hold you steady. When you feel anxious, angry, or upset, **STOP and feel your breathing**. Is it calm? Are you holding your breath? Is it racey? Now slow it down, just a little. Ahhh ... nice.

Hand breathing

Hold up your hand. With your pointer finger on the other hand, trace the outside of your hand. When you move up a finger, breathe in. Hold. When you move down, breathe out.

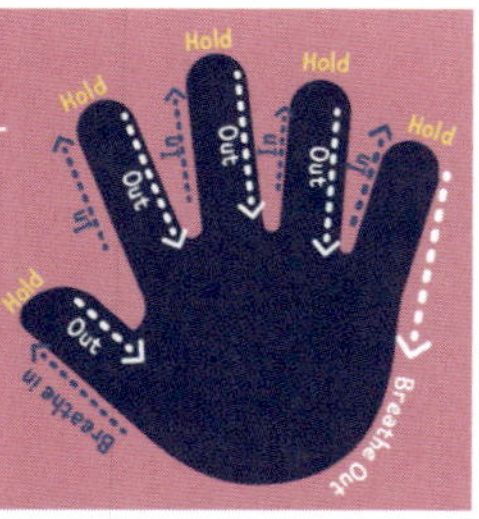

Butterfly breathing

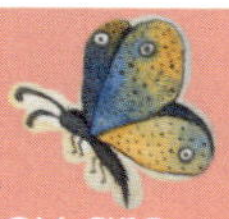

Breathe in for 3, raising your arms to the side, as though they are butterfly wings. As you lower them, breathe out slowly for 5, as though you're blowing out candles.

Hot cocoa breathing

Imagine holding a cup of hot cocoa in your hands. Breathe in the warm, chocolatey smell for 3, hold for 2, then gently blow on your cocoa to cool it for 5.

Sparkler breathing

Hold your hands down in front of you and imagine holding sparklers. Raise your arms out to the side then above you as you breathe in for 3. When your hands are above you, wave your sparklers and hold your breath for 2. Now, breathe out slowly for 5 as you take your sparklers back down and make the sound of sparklers hitting the water. Pssshhh

Figure 8 Breathing

Use your finger to trace a figure '8' on your skin. As you trace the first loop of the 8, breathe in for 3, hold in the middle for 1, breathe out for 3 as you trace the second loop of the 8.

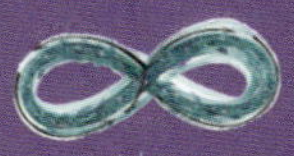

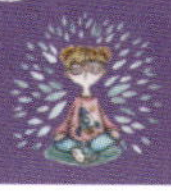

Dandelion breathing

Imagine where inside you your worries live. Imagine a big, fluffy dandelion there. Breathe in for 3. Hold for 1. As you breathe out for 5, imagine gently blowing the dandelion flowers away, as they carry your worries away with them.

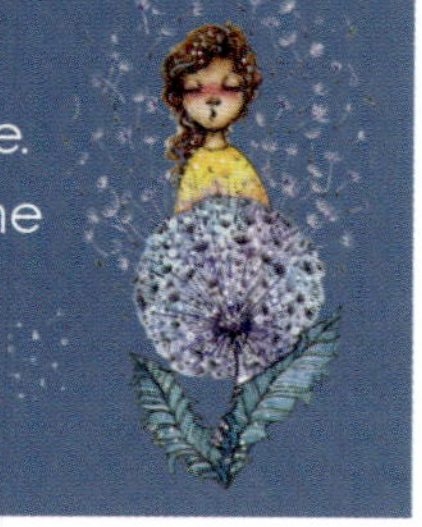

Belly breathing

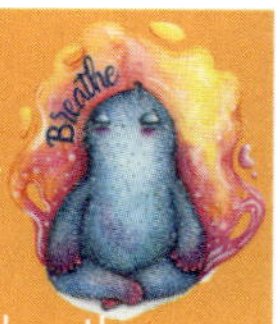

Sit back-to-back on the floor with a buddy. Let your backs touch, like you're holding each other up. Sit up tall, close your eyes (if you want), and start breathing slowly. Feel each other's backs move up and down - like a gentle little wave. Your breathing will start to match. Calm to calm.

Foggy window breathing

Breathe in, then as you exhale slowly, make a quiet 'ahhhh' noise as though you are fogging up a window.

Catch breathing

Take a deep breath in, hold it, then quickly inhale just a little more. Exhale slowly.

My amygdala loves ...

There are lots of different ways to calm anxiety. The right ones are the ones that feel right for *you*. Draw or write the ones you and your amygdala love most.

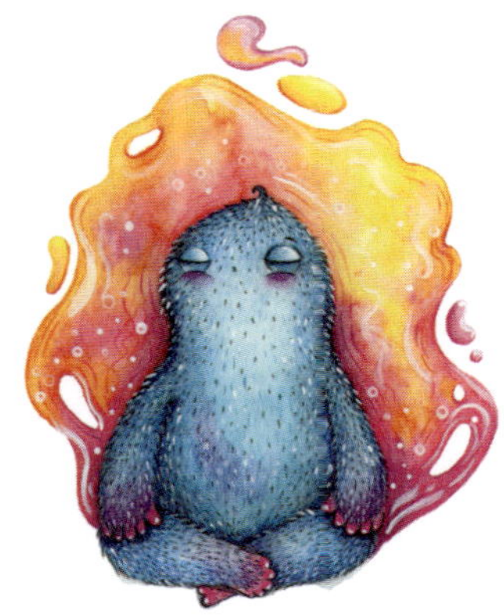

Something to remember ...

You are the most magnificent BRAIN BUILDER - and great things take time.

All these strategies might feel clunky at first - new things often do. That's not because you're doing them wrong or because they won't work. It's because your brain is still figuring them out. Keep going and you'll get the hang of them in no time. Are you with me? Phew. Because the party can't starty without you.

Here's why learning new things takes time: Your brain is made up of tiny building blocks called neurons. Everything you do depends on the pathways (the connections) between these neurons. This is how messages travel around your brain and body to tell your brain and body what to do. To do something well, you need the pathway to be clear and strong, so the messages can zoom around quickly.

When you try something new, like moving through the brave space, those neurons start chatting. As they do this, they build a pathway, like a pathway through the forest. At first, the pathway is bumpy and hard to see. It's as though your brain says, 'Hmmm, I'm not quite sure about this path. I don't know if I want to do this.'

The more you practice, the more the pathway gets used and the clearer it gets.

Eventually, when you've done that thing over and over, the pathway between the neurons gets clearer and stronger, and your brain goes, 'Oh I know this path! Let's do it!' This is when that thing you've been doing becomes easier or more automatic.

This is **'neuroplasticity'** — a fancy word that just means your brain can build and strengthen based on what you do. And you know who is in charge of this very incredible building process? You legend! It's you! Bit by bit. Step by step. Practice makes perfect ... pathways.

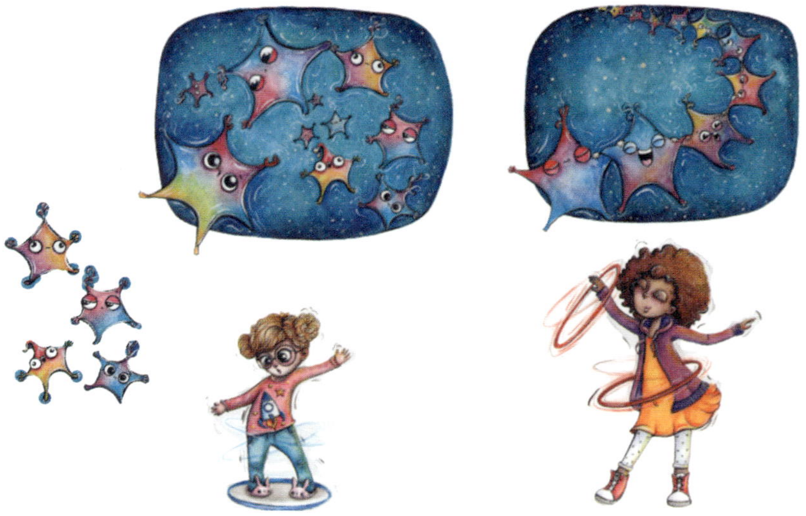

You already have strong pathways!

Write or draw the things you do well. Go for it!

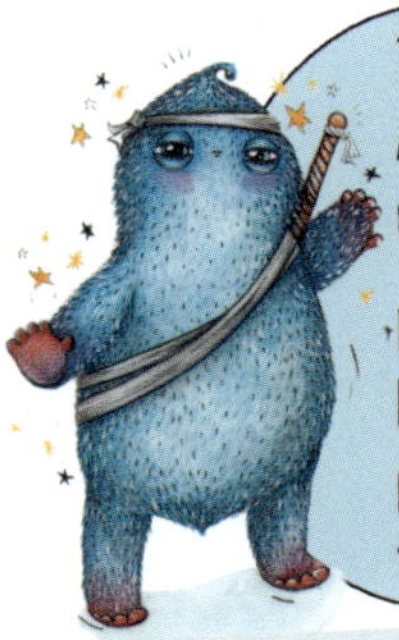

Think about the things you're good at – maybe drawing bugs, naming bugs (awww Albie – love that), running away from bugs, making bugs feel better about people running away, talking, or singing that song you sing (you know the one).

Now rewind. Was it always that way? Probably not. You're good at these things because you've done them a lot – maybe without noticing. Every time you did, the pathways in your brain got stronger and that thing got easier. There are loads of things you've become good at like this. What are some of them?

You're just getting started.

What brave, new, hard thing would you would like to get better at?

How can you build this pathway little by little? What's the first brave step?

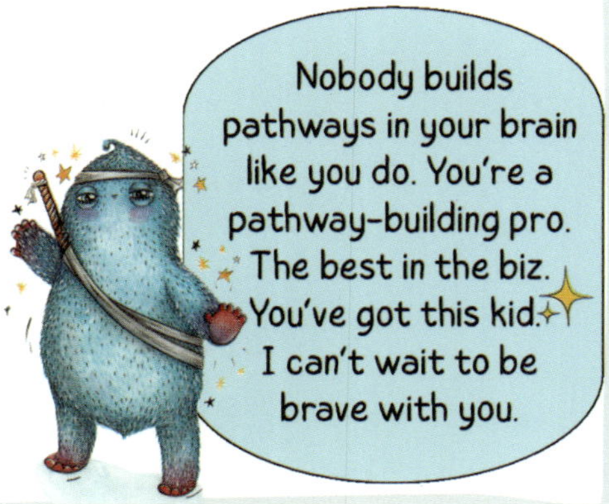

Also by Karen Young

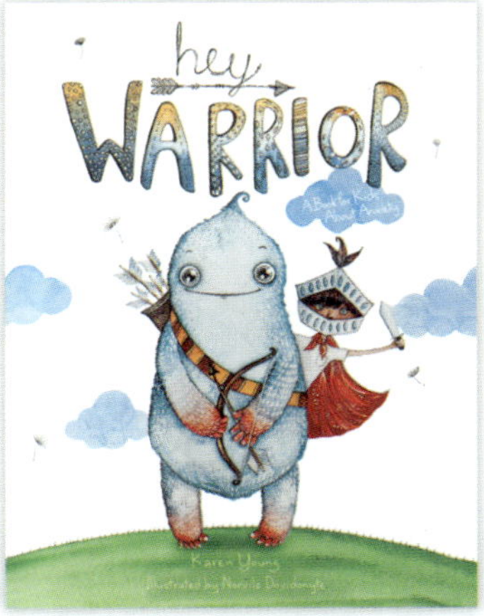

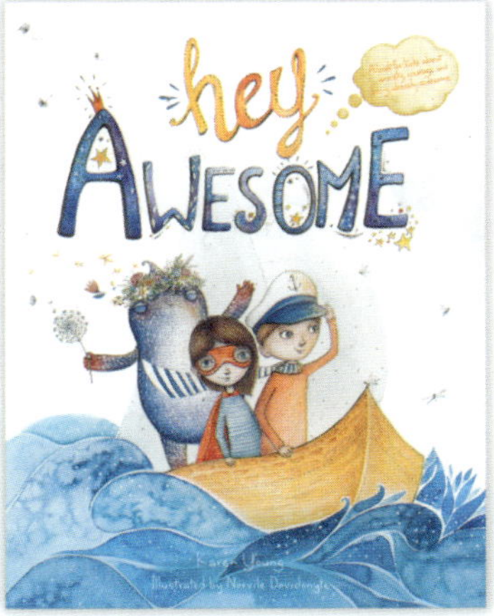

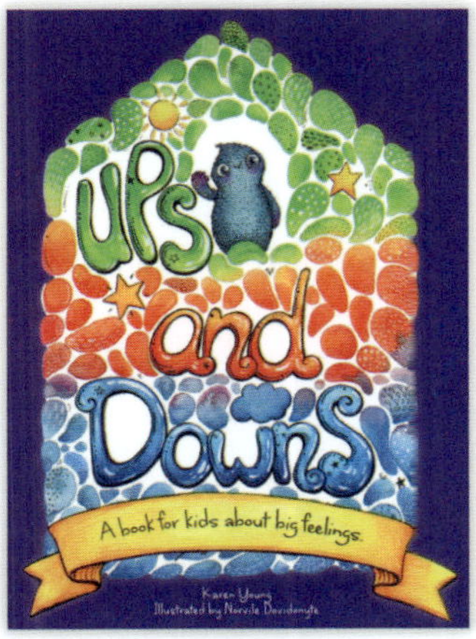

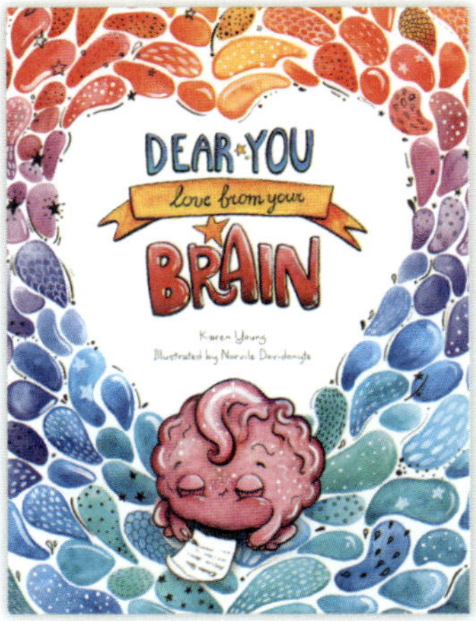

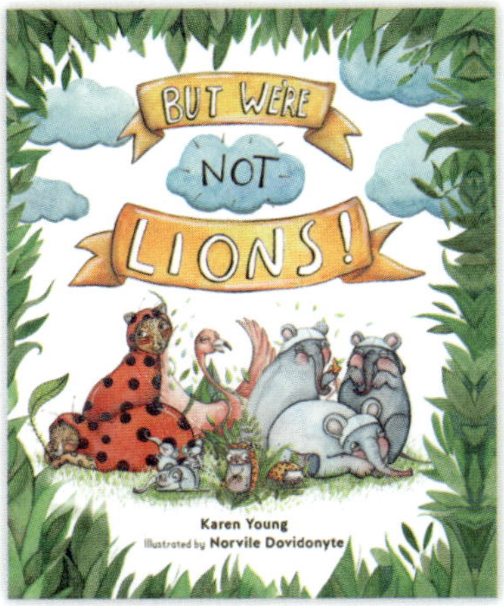

Published in Australia in 2025 by
Hey Sigmund Publishing, Brisbane.

www.heysigmund.com

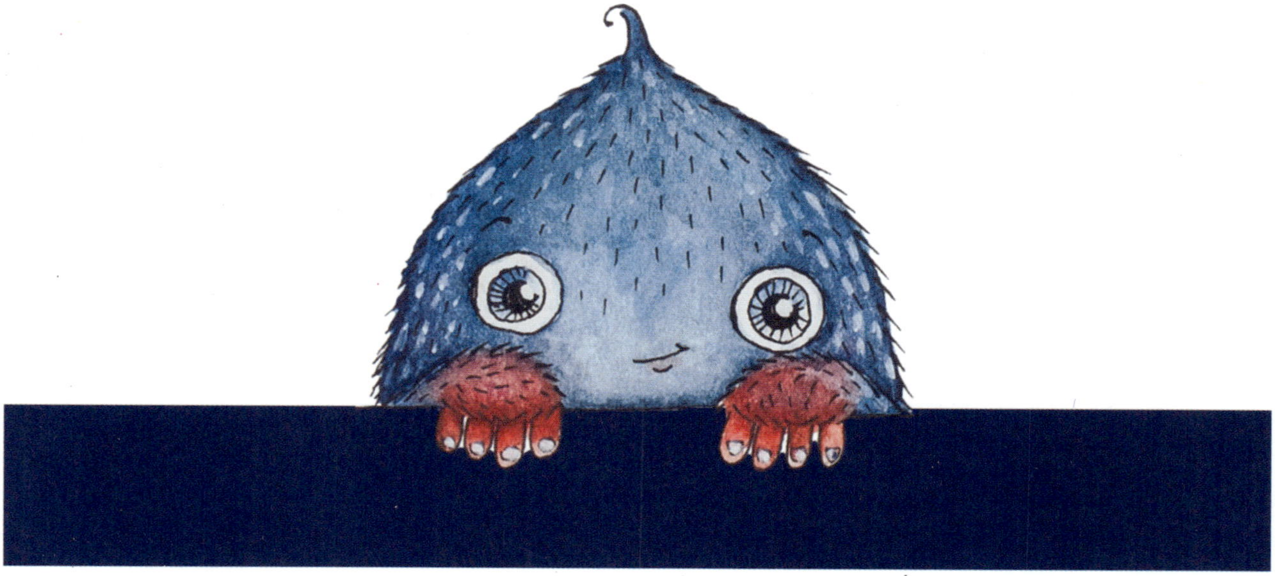